Tom-Louis W Gray Sr.

amaznut@yahoo.com

LOSE 30 POUNDS IN 90 DAYS WITH AMAZING SMOOTHIES RECIPES

by

Tom-Louis W Gray Sr.

Table of Contents

Improving Your Metabolism

TRYING TO FIND A WAY

Living a healthy life has become a great struggle here recently in America. There are so many things to learn about that it can become very confusing. Don't eat this! Don't eat that! Professionals in the medical field believe in one thing-holistic professionals believe in another. The stress that people feel in trying to live healthy can be overwhelming. Well there are simple ways. God designed our bodies to eat vegetables and water. We learn the system of getting our proteins from plant based foods because that where the animals that we eat get theirs. If there's any protein in chicken-the chicken got it from grains and other vegetation. The same philosophy goes for the Cow. Cows receive their protein from grazing in the field. That means that the protein is in the blood once that's cooked or dissolved there's no more protein. I know all of that may sound confusing but it's simple. "Eat vegetables and drink water.

You don't need to be a physique athlete to be serious about finding effective ways to get rid of body fat or live a healthy life. But just like a physique athlete you know that cutting your body's fat percentage is hard work and sometimes all it takes is for you to change WHAT YOU EAT! Hardly anyone has a perfect metabolism…one that automatically works to keep you in ideal form. Even if you do everything right to get leaner you may still struggle with your body fat percentages. Two metabolic factors are behind this huge problem.

The first factor is your body's ability to optimally produce thermogenic enzymes which create heat and burn calories. This is what the correct amount of protein consumption does to the human body cells. This condition may have not been a problem in your younger years but it gets worse as you grow older. If your metabolic rate is low and you begin a diet your (RMR) Resting Metabolic Rate diminishes even further causing frustration-confusion-fat gain and that ever so often recycling of new year resolutions. This will drive most people insane and mad as hell. This is what causes the YO-YO in weight gain-loss.

So as your great fitness nutrition coach I thought I'd share all of the Amazing Smoothies I have prepared for hundreds of faithful and loyal customers. It is part of my commitment and my assignment on earth to helping you all lose those unwanted pounds and inches. So if you're serious about finding an honest to goodness fat loss system or DIET then look no further. Because at Amazing Nutrition we have found a way to help you reach your fitness goals.

Amazing Smoothies!!!

Most people don't eat their five fruits and vegetables a day, or drink their eight cups of water. Smoothies simultaneously deliver one of each, which is far more convenient than drinking from a bottle of water while eating a piece of fruit with its requisite peels and juice.

Fruit smoothies deliver--particularly through blueberries--valuable antioxidants that boost your immune system.

Smoothies give you more energy by delivering carbohydrates that are less dense than more typical forms like bread and pasta.

Most adults don't regularly drink milk and instead get their dairy intake from cheese and butter, if they get it at all. Smoothies provide a painless way to drink milk every day, which helps muscle growth with its protein and bone strength with its calcium.

Fruit is a far better, more natural and a more efficient source of vitamins than those offered by supplements and pills. Smoothies are an excellent way to get your daily dose of vitamins.

Amazing Nutrition smoothies use only whole food ingredients-free of any artificial additives or synthetic sweeteners'. Our smoothies are 100% natural. Our smoothies are 70% organic and why would you need these things? To provide the necessary nutrients to achieve your performance or wellness goals. Amazing smoothies can be turned into a Low-Glycemic meal replacement for diabetic and bariatric patients also by adding a few healthy ingredients.

When people ask what's in my smoothies I reply "it's really what's not in them."

There is no Added Sugar-

There is no High Fructose Corn Syrup or processed Sugar.

There are No Preservatives or Additives of any kind

There are No Trans-Fats

There are No yellow or red dyes

There are No GMO's

There are No rBGH Hormones

Countless fat loss fads have come and gone in the last ten years. Some have been very dangerous and some just didn't pan out. Well Amazing Smoothies is not a fad. Actually you can do this forever from your own kitchen or office at anytime!! This is the real authentic Fast Food. Not Burgers and Fries or meals that are processed and filled with high amounts of chemicals and unhealthy additives. Processed foods eaten over periods of time keep your cells open which should not occur -then everything consumed by a person with open cells creates diseases such as diabetes-gout-arthritis-high blood pressure and many more. Smoothies that include whole and natural ingredients maintain the health of cells assuring that they open and close as they should. At Amazing Nutrition we want every calorie to be nutrient dense and naturally replete with the phyto-nutrients of whole foods necessary for rebuilding a new and better you!

What about the kids?

Parents are still feeding their precious babies hotdogs-potato chips and ice cream at birthday parties!

Kids need nutrition Too! Why? To provide the necessary nutrients to grow healthy. Here's a question I get all of the time and here's my answer. There isn't a child on earth that would turn down one of these smoothies. If they ask about the protein tell them that their cells are dividing at a faster rate than yours. Don't worry the 20 grams of protein is just what they need instead of a hotdog which may have 30 grams of nothing!!!!!

MYTH- Kids don't need protein.

WRONG! Your Kids cells are dividing and multiplying more rapidly than yours. Each cell is made with Amino Acids from protein.

MYTH- Protein will bulk me up!

WRONG- Your body needs protein to maintain healthy hair-nails-teeth-connective tissue-tendons-bones and a host other things that go on in the body.

MYTH- Women don't need as much protein as men!

WRONG- Active people need 1.5 grams of protein per body pound. Example (200 LB person) 200LB X 1.5grams = needs 300 grams protein per day for optimal body performance and nutrition.

Above are just a few myths that people have about proper nutrition. If you complete enough research you will find a bunch of truths about your nutrition.

<u>NUTRITION</u>

WHY IS NUTRITION IMPORTANT?

Nutrition: Just the Basics

Not only do what you eat affect your overall health, your diet will help you achieve all of your goals – whether you're aim is to build muscle or get lean. Food provides you the nutrients you need and also fuels your workouts. Before you take a dive into learning about nutrition for sports and exercise, it's important to understand the basics. Here are answers to frequently asked questions in my store:

Why is nutrition important?

On a fundamental level, nutrients are the building blocks of the body because they allow the body to grow and to repair itself. Healthy eating, which provides the nutrients your body needs, is essential to achieve peak performance in working out and in maintaining health. The concept of eating is big business! If you don't consider it that way then you are losing big time and headed for physical bankruptcy! You only eat to energize the body. If your (PA) is low or non-existent then you don't need the cow and the milk. This is when you have your smoothies to replace a meal. If you are going to run a marathon then you need a large amount of protein and carbohydrates.

What are nutrients?

There are six major classes of nutrients: water, carbohydrate, fat, protein, vitamins, and minerals.

Water: The body is made of as much as 75% water. Staying hydrated is essential for basic physiological actions inside the body, including digestion and absorption of the food and nutrients you consume.

Carbs: Carbohydrates help provide energy—as calories—for fueling your workouts, and many carbohydrate containing foods also provide fiber to keep your gastrointestinal tract healthy.

Fat: Fat provides energy and is essential for transportation and absorption of some vitamins in the body. Stored fat helps protect organs and maintain body temperature.

Protein: Protein provides energy and is involved with your immune system and with enzymes that drive chemical reactions in the body.

Vitamins and Minerals: Without providing caloric energy, vitamins and minerals perform numerous roles, including keeping bones healthy, helping in fuel metabolism, serving as antioxidants that may help ward off chronic illnesses, and helping the blood clot properly.

Bottom line: the food you put into your body determines how healthy you will be and how you function during your workouts. Furthermore, no amount of exercise will compensate for a poor diet.

How much do I need?

This is highly variable depending upon your unique nutritional needs. General health status, activity levels, lifestyle, age, and biological sex are some of many determinants of optimal nutrition. In general, a healthful diet comprises mostly unrefined, whole grain carbohydrates (e.g., oats, whole wheat, brown rice, quinoa), lean proteins (i.e., chicken breast), unsaturated fats (i.e., vegetable oils and foods made with vegetable oils, and nut oils), and as many fruits and vegetables as desired.

You are WHAT YOU EAT!

Fueling for Carbohydrates Performance

Whether you're trying to build muscle or trying to burn fat or get lean and toned, you may have questions about how carbohydrates (AKA, carbs) fit into your diet. Here are some frequently asked questions and answers to carbohydrate questions I've answered in consultations.

Why do I need carbs?

Along with protein and fat, carbohydrates are essential macronutrients that give you energy. In fact, studies show that having adequate carbohydrate stores will help you stave off fatigue, perform better and get the most out of your workout as you push the intensity and duration. Your body stores carbs as glycogen (chains of glucose molecules) in the liver and in the muscles. Your glycogen stores provide quick, efficient energy, especially for high-intensity exercise (explosive, powerful movements). Basically, carbohydrates are the major, "high-octane fuel sources" for exercise. Some famous doctor created a low carb diet which fooled so many people for a long time! I used to get approached by individuals in the health clubs and they would ask that famous question " How can I build more muscle? My answer would be a simple increase your protein and carbohydrate consumption! Then I would get the fabulous I don't want to offend anybody response "I thought carbs made you fat and I don't want to be a big muscle bodybuilder!!!!! Nonsense! So check out below how many carbohydrates should be in your diet for optimal efficiency.

How much do I need?

The amount of carbohydrates you need to eat on a daily basis will depend on your activity level and typically ranges from 2.7 to 4.5 grams per pound for athletes. A sports dietitian can assess your unique needs and provide you with a personalized recommendation. In general, the daily carbohydrate requirements based on how often and how hard you workout are moderate intensity and duration of activity, 2-3 times/week: ~2-3 grams per pound of body weight

Higher intensity and duration of activity, 4-6 times/week: ~4-5 grams per pound of body weight

When should I eat Carbohydrates?

Before a workout

Eating before a workout – especially carbohydrates – will help improve your performance. The goal is to have a meal or snack that tops off your fuel stores, but doesn't leave you hungry nor with a full belly. Research shows that a carb-rich meal (~200-300 grams) about 3-4 hours prior to exercise will optimally enhance performance. In addition to consuming adequate carbs, here are other pre-workout helpful hints:

Pass on slow-to-digest fatty and high-fiber foods

Enjoy familiar carbohydrate/moderate protein foods and beverages to avoid gastrointestinal discomfort.

Try a liquid carbohydrate source, such as an Amazing Smoothie or beverages if your stomach doesn't tolerate solid foods.

To top off stores before a competition or challenging workout, have a high carb snack 30-60 minutes before you start

During a workout

Studies show that consuming carbs during a workout can help you maintain your blood sugar (glucose) levels and improve performance. The amount of carbohydrates that you need during a workout depends on the duration of the workout.

<u>If you're working out for less than 60 min:</u> Some research shows that consuming carbs from a sports drink (6-8% carb sports drink) may help improve performance, especially if you're exercising on empty after an overnight fast. <u>For over an hour:</u> every 15-20 minutes consume carbs for a total of 30-60 grams of per hour to extend endurance performance

After a workout

Right after you exercise, your body is ready to recover and replenish glycogen stores. Follow these three simple steps:

1. Eat as soon as possible after exercise (within 30 min).

2. Get a combination of carbohydrate and protein: 2-3 grams of carbs for every 1 gram of protein. Example (25 grams of protein -75 grams of Carbohydrates. This is not appropriate for those that participate in classic cardio. Classic Cardio is sitting on a stationary bike/walking on a treadmill/or gliding on an ski machine for 60 minutes or more. These people will continue to gain fat and we see them every day at the health club. Classic Cardio does not raise the heart enough to burn fat.

3. Eat a meal or consume an Amazing Smoothie every 2-3 hours or so to maximize glycogen stores. Below are examples of carbohydrates to consume.

What foods have 25-30 grams of carbs?

1 cup juice or 1 large piece of fruit-1 small bagel or 2 slices of bread

1 cup of most cereals-1 large baked potato

2 cups of milk-1 cup of rice or corn

2 cups of sports drink- to 1 energy bar, depending on the brand

<u>WORKOUT RECOVERY FOODS AND DRINKS</u>

TIMING IS EVERYTHING

Recover Right

Sports nutrition experts agree that what you do *after* a workout is just as important as what you do *during* a workout. Proper recovery nutrition is the key to realizing your goals and reaping the benefits from your workout. Replenishing and refueling supports muscle growth and repair, helps to decrease core temperature, replaces muscle carbohydrate stores (glycogen), rehydrates and will help you take your performance to the next level. Here are some frequently asked questions and answers about recovery that I give to my clients and customers.

Why do I need to eat after a workout?

After you workout, your insulin levels are low, leptin levels are low, stress hormones are elevated, muscle and liver glycogen has gone down, muscle breakdown is increased, and fuel and fluid levels are likely depleted. Left unattended, this post-exercise environment can lead to increased muscle soreness, extended fatigue and low energy. It is very dangerous to continue this behavior over time. You practically just wasted a workout! In order to avoid these consequences and enhance performance, recovery nutrition is a priority.

By eating after your workout, you can turn the body's post-exercise responses into gains.

Recovery eating:

Increases blood insulin

Lowers stress hormone levels

Restores muscle and liver glycogen

Slows muscle breakdown and promotes protein synthesis

Refuels and rehydrates

Makes you harder and leaner

When should I eat and drink for recovery?

Your body is ready to recover and replenish glycogen stores immediately after you exercise. Don't miss this window of opportunity – try to eat within 30 minutes of finishing your workout (15-30 grams of protein and 40-80 grams of carbohydrates) and again in 2 to 3 hours to maximize glycogen replacement.

What should I eat?

For both endurance and strength workouts, carbohydrates and protein are the macronutrients you need and fluids will help you rehydrate:

Carbohydrates: 0.5-3.0 grams/kilogram body weight carbohydrate/or per gram of protein

Protein: 20-25 grams protein

Fluid/water should be replaced at 2 to 3 cups per every pound of body weight lost during exercise (measure your body weight pre-exercise for comparison)

Body weight LB / 2.2 X 0.5 = grams of carbohydrates; body weight LB / 2.2 X 1.0 = grams of carbohydrates:

Examples of 25-30 grams of carbs to eat after a workout.

1 cup juice or 1 large piece of fruit

1 small bagel or 2 slices of bread

2 cups of milk

1 cup of rice or corn

2 cups of sports drink-Lite Powder and Ready-to-Drink protein supplements.

Examples of 20-25 grams of protein

3 eggs, 6 egg whites

2 cups of milk

¾ cup of cottage cheese

3 cups of yogurt

3 oz. chicken, fish, pork or beef

3 oz. of cheese (except cream cheese)

6 T. peanut butter

24 oz. soy milk

Protein drinks and powders (typically 10-45 g/serving)

WHICH SMOOTHIE SHOULD I DRINK & WHY?

Basically all of the smoothies can be used for recovery because they all have nutrient dense carbohydrates as their foundation but each smoothie has outstanding benefits. One may do a better job than another based on the level and ratio of macros (protein-carbs-fats). No calorie is empty therefore no calorie is wasted. Your job is to figure out which smoothie is the best smoothie for you at that moment in time.

Whether your goal is burning fat-building muscle or both your body will always use glycogen first even if you are in an oxidative state.

Glycogen is stored sugar held in your muscle fibers and liver. This "sugar" was previously carbohydrates broken down by your body from fruit-veggies-grains-beans and legumes. Because you have used most or all of your glycogen (stored carbs) during your workout your body requires restoring its glycogen to pre-workout levels. This is Key. If your body doesn't receive the necessary carbohydrates from easily digestible sources (blended whole foods) it will begin breaking down your hard earned muscle tissue and turning muscle into sugar and then into glycogen to refill its glycogen stores. This is called Gluconeogenisis or more commonly a Catabolic State. Bad! Ultimately this burns off muscle and holds onto your fat increasing your fat to muscle ratio and decreasing your metabolic rate! So bad yet soooooo many people do this simply by drinking only water after a workout.

All smoothies will refuel depleted glycogen stores if consumed within 30 minutes of a workout. This should be your primary objective after a workout and the most important meal of the day. Remember calories consumed immediately after a workout are not stored as fat but instead those calories Refuel-Replenish- and Revolumize MUSCLE cells. These are free calories and they complete a workout.

All of these smoothies are approximately the same amount of calories-about 400 with a perfect 3/1 ratio of carbohydrates/protein. Each smoothie has 20 grams of whey protein added so that muscle can be rebuilt one cell at a time with much needed amino acids.

THESE ARE THE AMAZING SMOOTHIES

Egg Nog

Low Fat Organic Egg Nog-1 Scoop Vanilla Protein

Green Nut

4 oz of Vanilla Almond Milk-teaspoon Matcha Green Tea-1 Scoop of Pistachios-1 scoop of Vanilla Protein- Honey or Agave.

Sweet Potato Pie

1 scoop Vanilla Protein-Potato Puree- Chia Tea-Cinnamon-Vanilla Extract-Honey

Apple Pie

1 scoop Vanilla Protein-4 Apple pieces- (1) tablespoon Chia Tea- 1 teaspoon Cinnamon

Peach Cobbler

1 scoop Vanilla Protein-4 peach pieces-(1) tablespoon of Chia Tea-1 teaspoon Cinnamon

Strawberry Nana

4 Strawberry pieces, ½ Banana & 1 scoop Vanilla Whey Protein.

Amazing Brew

Water, Soy or Almond Milk, 1 scoop Instant Coffee, 1 scoop Chocolate & Vanilla Whey Protein.

Mango Madness

8 pieces/Mangoes, ¼ Banana, 4 pieces Strawberries/Pineapple & 1 scoop Vanilla Whey Protein.

Hawaiian Hulu

8 pieces/Pineapple, ½ Banana, scoop of Coconut & Vanilla Whey Protein.

Berry Good Berries

4 pieces each Raspberries, Blackberries Strawberries, 8/Blueberries, ¼ Banana & scoop of Vanilla Whey Protein.

Chocolate Mint

Water, Soy or Almond Milk, Chocolate, Mint, Chocolate Whey Protein

Banana Nut Bread

(1) Banana, 1 tlbs. Almond Butter, Water, or 4 oz. Almond Milk & Vanilla Whey Protein.

Peanut Butter Delight

1 scoop Chocolate, 1 tblsp Peanut Butter, Water, Soy or 4 oz Almond Milk & 1 scoop Chocolate Whey Protein.

Texas Trail Mix

1 tblsp Almond Butter, Water, Soy or 4 oz Almond Milk, scoop Cinnamon Granola, ¼ Banana, Raisins & Vanilla Whey Protein.

Black Tie

4 oz Almond or Soy Milk-scoop Chia Tea- scoop Chocolate Protein & Vanilla Protein

Blues Blaster

8 blueberry Pieces-1/2 Banana-1 scoop Vanilla Protein-

Super Builder

4 oz Almond or Soy Milk- scoop Vanilla or Chocolate Protein-1 scoop Creatine-Banana

Chocolate Frosty

Chocolate Almond Milk-1 scoop of Nestle Chocolate-1 scoop Chocolate Protein

Chocolate Butter Peel

Chocolate Almond Milk-1 Banana-1 scoop Chocolate Protein-1 tblsp Peanut Butter

Go Green

6 Pineapple pieces- ½ Banana-4 oz Kale -Vanilla Protein

Green Machine

6 Pineapple pieces ½ Banana-1 scoop Vanilla Protein-1 scoop low fat Yogurt-Spinach or

kale

Lime Light

8 Lime pieces-1 Banana-1 scoop Vanilla Protein

Muscle Mass

4 oz Almond or Soy Milk-1 scoop Chocolate Protein-1/2 Banana- 1 scoop Oatmeal- 1 tblsp

Almond Butter

Lemonana

4 Lemon pieces-1 Banana-1 scoop Vanilla Protein

Trix

2 Lemon pieces- 4 Strawberries-1 Bananas-1 scoop Vanilla Protein

Tropical Fruit

4 Strawberries-1 Bananas-4 Pineapples pieces- 1 scoop Vanilla Protein-

Mocha & Latte Licious

Vanilla Almond Milk-1 scoop Vanilla Protein-1 scoop Mocha- 1 scoop Latte Coffee

Vanilla Charm

1 scoop Vanilla Protein-4 oz Vanilla Almond Milk- 1 Banana

Banana Slim

4 oz Almond or Soy Milk-1 scoop Vanilla Protein-1 Banana

Berry Trim

8 Blueberry Pieces-4 Strawberries-1 scoop Vanilla Protein-4 oz Vanilla Almond Milk

Tom's 6 Pack Attack

4 oz Skim Milk-1 scoop Chocolate- Chocolate Protein-1/4 Banana

Energize Me

4 Orange pieces-4 small Carrots -1/4 Banana-1 oz Beet juice -1 scoop Vanilla Protein

Lean Machine

4 oz Water-1 scoop Vanilla Protein-1/2 Banana-1 scoop Glutamine

Mango-Licious

8 Mango pieces-2 Orange pieces-1 scoop Vanilla Protein-1/4 Banana

Green Tea Lite

4 oz Water-1 scoop Vanilla Protein-1/4 Banana-1 scoop Matcha Green Tea

PB Cup Lite

4 oz Skim Milk-1 scoop Chocolate Choice-1 scoop Chocolate Protein-1 tblsp Almond Butter

Pina Cream

8 Pineapple pieces-1 scoop Vanilla Protein-1 scoop shredded Coconut

Skinny Tommy

4 oz Skim Milk-1/4 Banana-1 tblsp Almond Butter-1 scoop Vanilla Protein

Strawberry Slim

8 Strawberries pieces-choice of (Orange Lemon or Lime) 1/2 Bananas-1 scoop Vanilla Protein

Almond Joy

4 oz Vanilla Almond Milk-Scoop of Coconut-Scoop (8) Almonds-1 scoop Chocolate Protein.

Instructions for Weight Loss

1

Choose your ingredients. There are a multitude of foods that you can use to make a smoothie. The basics are low fat milk, low fat vanilla yogurt Almond milk and a handful of ice. Once you have those, you can add bananas, cantaloupe, peanut butter, strawberries, or anything that sounds good.

2

Make your smoothie. This example is called the Banana Split smoothie. You need 1 banana, 1 6 oz. cup of low fat vanilla yogurt, 1/8 cup of frozen orange juice, 1/2 cup low fat milk/or Almond Milk , 2scp. vanilla whey protein powder and 6 crushed ice cubes. Blend it using the pulse button until you get the consistency you want. This will make enough for two meals so you have something to take on the go with you if need be. Preparation time is a mere five minutes.

3

Drink your lunch. Enjoy the remainder of the smoothie you made from breakfast for your lunch. This should do the trick until you get home. If you need a snack, be sure to keep a piece of fruit or some nuts on hand to snack on in between. For best results purchase a small personal blender for your office or at school. A smoothie at 6am-9am-12noon-and

3pm will provide you with 4 meals. You can then eat a sensible dinner around 6pm and a healthy snack before bedtime. Your metabolism will turn into an inferno!!!!!

4

Eat a healthy dinner. Smoothies are great meal replacement options, but you still need to eat at least one regular meal a day. This can be any meal that is of the most convenience to you and your schedule, so interchange this according to your schedule.

5

Enjoy a snack. Rather than eating a bowl of ice cream before bed, make another smoothie. It's just as tasty, it's more filling and definitely healthier. In addition, you will always get two servings whenever you prepare your smoothies, so you can store your leftovers for another meal or for another snack.

Enjoy Your Healthy Living!

www.ingramcontent.com/pod-product-compliance
Lightning Source LLC
Chambersburg PA
CBHW081152290526

45795CB00008B/2896